LOW CARB
EGG COOKBOOK

49 Mouthwatering Low Carb Egg Recipes for Quick, Easy and Healthy Weight Loss!

ATHAR HUSAIN

Panjtan Publication House

PLEASE ALWAYS KEEP IN TOUCH WITH ME TO UPDATE YOURSELF WITH MY BOOKS.

EMAIL Athar Husain at--atharhusain2015@gmail.com

Also by- Athar Husain:

50 MOUTHWATERING LOW CARB RECIPES FOR RAPID WEIGHT LOSS!

http://www.amazon.com/CARB-RECIPES-WEIGHT-LOSS-MOUTHWATERING-ebook/dp/B00XCRET4Q/

50 Incredibly delicious low carb recipes for fast and healthy

Weight loss!

http://www.amazon.com/gp/product/B01047HHAY

INTRODUCTION

Thank you for downloading the copy of, **"49 Mouthwatering Low Carb Egg Recipes for Quick, Easy and Healthy Weight Loss!"**

Inside this Cook Book you will find 49 delicious and mouthwatering **Low Carb Egg recipes** that you'll definitely love. If you want to eat healthy and lose weight rapidly then this low carb Egg Cook Book is for you.

If you take foods with high carbohydrates, you are under the high risk of **Diabetes type-2, excessive and rapid weight gain.** It is advisable to take only **low carb healthy foods**. In busy schedule, people don't have much time to spend in the kitchen and they easily adopt poor eating habit. But you don't worry about time because most of the recipes take **only 30 min or less to cook** inside this cook book.

As everybody knows that **Eggs are the rich source of protein** and **protein are very essential for human body.** You can add eggs in your food because **Eggs are less expensive** and easily available and delicious in taste too. So if you **trying to lose some excess pounds** then you should definitely eat low carb egg recipe in your breakfast, lunch or dinner.

The foods are **simple to cook and delicious** in taste too. I have included nutritional information with each recipes to help you with your weight loss goals. Inside this book I have included **49 Mouthwatering Low Carb Egg Recipes that you will definitely love.**

All these recipes are very yummy and easy to cook. Reason, behind the popularity of Low-Carb Diet is that, it helps to **reduce weight** and also help to **prevent Diabetes, cardiovascular disease and high Blood Pressure.**

This Book contains **Delicious Breakfast, Lunch, Dinner, Appetizers, Snacks and Desserts... Egg Recipes in one pack.** So just discard your old boring low carb recipes cook book and try this mouthwatering Low-Carb recipes book today.

Just click on the hyperlink of your favorite recipe from the table of content and start enjoying your Low Carb Egg Recipe while losing weight!

Here we start the journey to weight loss while remain healthy.......

TABLE OF CONTENT

DINNER EGG RECIPES

APPETIZERS

SNACKS

DESSERTS

BREAKFAST EGG RECIPES

#1. Devilled Eggs with Dill Recipe

Total Prepare/ Cook Time: - 20 min.

Servings: 6

Ingredients:

6 eggs (hard and cooked)

2 tablespoons Mayonnaise (Low-Fat)

1-1/2 teaspoon cider vinegar

3/4 teaspoon mustard

1/4 teaspoon salt

1/4 teaspoon Worcestershire sauce

Small amount of pepper

12 dill springs, fresh

Instructions:

1. Cut eggs in equal halves. Remove egg yolks from four eggs and put aside.

2. Take a large bowl and mash the yolks. Mix in the vinegar, mustard, mayonnaise, Worcestershire sauce, pepper and salt. Put into white eggs. Garnish with dill.

3. Place into the refrigerator until serving.

Nutritional information per serving:

Calories: 74

Fat: 5g

Protein: 5g

Carbohydrates: 1g

#2. Eggs in Foil Bowls Recipe

Total Prepare/ Cook Time: - 30 min.

Servings: 3

Ingredients:

6 eggs

1/3 cup milk

1/8 teaspoon salt

1/8 teaspoon pepper

1/8 teaspoon garlic powder

1/4 cup green pepper, finely chopped

1/2 cup cheddar cheese, shredded

4 fully cooked breakfast sausage links, frozen and chopped

4 fully cooked bacon strips, crumbled

2 green onions, finely chopped

Instructions:

1. Firstly prepare grill then take a small bowl. Mix eggs, milk, salt, pepper and garlic powder properly.

2. Grease a medium pan with cooking spray and pour the prepared mixture into the pan.

3. Now drizzle with cheese, sausage, bacon, green pepper and onions.

4. Now cover up the pan with foil and grill for about 20-30 minutes or until the eggs are completely cook.

Nutritional information per serving:

Calories: 346

Fat: 26g

Protein: 23g

Carbohydrates: 5g

#3. Sausage, Eggs and Cheddar Recipe

Total Prepare/ Cook Time: - 20 min.

Servings: 4

Ingredients:

6 eggs

1/3 cup milk

1/2 teaspoon parsley flakes, dried

1/4 teaspoon salt

6 oz. bulk pork sausage

1-1/2 cups frozen mash brown potatoes, thawed

1/4 cup onion, finely chopped

4 oz. cheddar cheese, cut into pieces

Instructions:

1. Beat the eggs, parsley, milk and salt well and put aside. Take a large frying pan and cook sausage over medium heat then take out from pan and drain it.

2. In the same frying pan cook onion and potatoes for 6-7 minutes then again put the sausage into pan.

3. Add egg mixture and cook it properly. Drizzle with cheese. Again cook for 2-3 minutes or until cheese melted.

Nutritional information per serving:

Calories: 330

Fat: 24g

Protein: 20g

Carbohydrates: 9g

#4. Quick Fluffy Scrambled Eggs Recipe

Total Prepare/ Cook Time: - 15 min.

Servings: 4

Ingredients:

8 eggs

5 oz. evaporated milk

2 tablespoons butter

1/2 teaspoon salt

Small amount of pepper

Instructions:

1. Take a medium bowl and beat the eggs and milk properly.

2. Take a large frying pan and heat up the butter. Add egg mixture and cook for 8-10 minutes over medium heat or until the eggs cooked properly.

3. Drizzle with salt and pepper. Enjoy you quick fluffy scrambled egg recipe.

Nutritional information per serving:

Calories: 244

Fat: 18g

Protein: 15g

Carbohydrates: 5g

#5. Baked Omelet Roll Recipe

Total Prepare/ Cook Time: - 30 min.

Servings: 6

Ingredients:

6 eggs

1 cup milk

1/2 teaspoon salt

1/2 cup all-purpose flour

4 oz. cheddar cheese, cut into pieces

1/4 teaspoon pepper

Instructions:

1. Mix eggs, milk, flour, salt and pepper in the blender and blend until smooth.

2. Grease a large baking pan and pour the mixture into pan. Bake for 20-25 minutes at 375 Fahrenheit.

3. Drizzle with cheese then roll up the omelet in pan.

4. Enjoy the delicious baked omelet roll this morning.

Nutritional information per serving:

Calories: 204

Fat: 12g

Protein: 13g

Carbohydrates: 10g

#6. Scrambled Egg Muffins Recipe

Total Prepare/ Cook Time: - 30 min.

Servings: 12

Ingredients:

12 eggs

1/2 lbs. bulk pork sausage

1/2 cup onion, finely chopped

1/4 cup green pepper, finely chopped

1/4 teaspoon garlic powder

1/2 teaspoon salt

1/4 teaspoon pepper

1/2 cup cheddar cheese, cut into pieces

Instructions:

1. Heat up the oven to 350 Fahrenheit. Take a large frying pan and cook sausage over medium heat.

2. Beat eggs in a large bowl and add onion, salt, green pepper, garlic powder and pepper. Mix with spoon into sausage and cheese.

3. Coated muffin cups with cooking spray and put the egg mixture into muffin cups and bake for 20-25 minutes.

Nutritional information per serving:

Calories: 133

Fat: 10g

Protein: 9g

Carbohydrates: 2g

#7. Baked Eggs with Cheddar and Bacon Recipe

Total Prepare/ Cook Time: - 25 min.

Servings: 4

Ingredients:

4 eggs

4 tablespoons milk, (Fat-Free)

2 tablespoons cheddar cheese, cut into pieces

2 teaspoons fresh parsley, crumbled

1/8 teaspoon pepper

1/4 teaspoon salt

2 bacon strips

Instructions:

1. Heat up the oven to 350 Fahrenheit. Grease 4 ounce ramekins with cooking spray.

2. Now break an egg and put into each dish. Pour 1 tablespoon milk over each egg.

3. Mix cheese, pepper, parsley and salt and drizzle over it.

4. Bake for 13-15 minutes. At the same time cook bacon over medium heat in a small frying pan. Take out bacon and drain.

5. Cut the bacon into pieces and drizzle over eggs.

Nutritional information per serving:

Calories: 107

Fat: 7g

Protein: 9g

Carbohydrates: 1g

#8. Vegetable Scrambled Eggs Recipe

Total Prepare/ Cook Time: - 15 min.

Servings: 2

Ingredients:

4 eggs

1/2 cup green pepper, finely chopped

1/4 cup green onions, thinly sliced

1/4 cup milk

1/8 teaspoon pepper

1/2 teaspoon salt

1 medium tomato, finely chopped

Instructions:

1. Take a small bowl and mix eggs, milk, green pepper, onions, pepper and salt.

2. Grease the medium frying pan and pour the mixture into it. Cook over medium heat.

3. Now add tomato and cook until the eggs cooked properly.

4. Enjoy the delicious vegetable scrambled eggs with your family.

Nutritional information per serving:

Calories: 96

Fat: 0g

Protein: 14g

Carbohydrates: 9g

#9. Cheesy Chive Omelet Recipe

Total Prepare/ Cook Time: - 15 min.

Servings: 2

Ingredients:

3 eggs

2 tablespoons water

1/8 teaspoon salt

Small amount of pepper

1 tablespoon butter

1 tablespoon fresh chives, crumbled

1/2 cup cheddar cheese, cut into pieces

Instructions:

1. Take a small bowl and beat eggs, water, pepper and salt. Mix with spoon in chives.

2. Take a small frying pan and heat butter over medium heat. Put into egg mixture.

3. Push egg's cooked portion toward the center and uncooked eggs flow underneath.

4. When the eggs cooked completely. Drizzle cheese only one side. Fold and cut the omelet in half.

5. Don't forget to add this yummy recipe in your breakfast.

Nutritional information per serving:

Calories: 216

Fat: 18g

Protein: 13g

Carbohydrates: 1g

#10. Spinach-Mushroom Scrambled Eggs Recipe

Total Prepare/ Cook Time: - 15 min.

Servings: 2

Ingredients:

2 large eggs with white

1/8 teaspoon pepper

1/8 teaspoon salt

1 teaspoon butter

1/2 cup fresh mushrooms, thinly sliced

1/2 cup fresh baby spinach, finely chopped

2 tablespoon provolone cheese, cut into pieces

Instructions:

1. Beat eggs, egg whites, pepper and salt in a small bowl. Take a small frying pan and heat butter over medium heat.

2. Add mushrooms and cook for 4-5 minutes. Then add spinach and cook over medium heat.

3. Add egg mixture and cook until eggs cooked completely. Mix with spoon in cheese.

4. Enjoy this delicious low carb egg recipe in the breakfast

Nutritional information per serving:

Calories: 162

Fat: 11g

Protein: 14g

Carbohydrates: 2g

.

LUNCH EGG RECIPES

#11. Eggs with Bacon Recipe

Total Prepare/ Cook Time: - 30 min.

Servings: 24

Ingredients:

12 eggs (hard-cooked)

1/3 cup mayonnaise

3 cooked bacon strips, crumbled

3 tablespoons red onion, finely chopped

3 tablespoons sweet pickle relish

1/4 teaspoon smoked paprika

Instructions:

1. Cut the eggs into halves and take out yolks. Mash yolks in a small bowl.

2. Mix bacon, mayonnaise, onion and relish very well. Put into egg whites.

3. Put into refrigerator until serving. Drizzle with paprika.

4. Enjoy the yummy Deviled Eggs with Bacon with your family.

Nutritional information per serving:

Calories: 68

Fat: 5g

Protein: 3g

Carbohydrates: 1g

#12. No-Yolk Eggs Recipe

Total Prepare/ Cook Time: - 20 min.

Servings: 10

Ingredients:

10 eggs (hard-cooked)

3/4 cup potatoes, mashed

1 tablespoon mayonnaise (Fat-Free)

1 teaspoon mustard

Small amount of yellow food coloring

Paprika

Instructions:

1. Cut eggs into slices and remove yolks.

2. Mix mashed potatoes, mustard, mayonnaise and food coloring thoroughly in a small bowl.

3. Put the stuff into egg whites. Drizzle with paprika. Put into refrigerator till serving.

Nutritional information per serving:

Calories: 35

Fat: 1g

Protein: 4g

Carbohydrates: 3g

#13. Cream Cheese Egg Recipe

Total Prepare/ Cook Time: - 25 min.

Servings: 16

Ingredients:

8 large eggs (hard-cooked)

8 oz. softened cream cheese

1/4 teaspoon pepper

2 teaspoons Dijon mustard

1/4 teaspoon salt

1/4 cup frozen peas, drain

3 cooked bacon strips, crumbled

Instructions:

1. Cut eggs into slices and remove yolks.

2. Mash yolks in a small bowl and mix mustard, cream cheese, pepper and salt then beat until smooth. Mix with spoon in peas.

3. Put the stuff into egg whites. Drizzle with bacon. Put into refrigerator till serving.

Nutritional information per serving:

Calories: 97

Fat: 8g

Protein: 5g

Carbohydrates: 1g

#14. Delightful Deviled Eggs Recipe

Total Prepare/ Cook Time: - 20 min.

Servings: 6

Ingredients:

6 large eggs (hard-cooked)

1-1/2 teaspoon grated onion

2 tablespoons mayonnaise

1-1/2 teaspoon sweet pickle relish

1/2 teaspoon spicy brown mustard

1/8 teaspoon pepper

1/8 teaspoon red pepper flakes, crushed

1/4 teaspoon salt

Instructions:

1. Cut the eggs into halves and take out yolks. Mash yolks in a small bowl. Mix with spoon in the mayonnaise, relish, onion, mustard, pepper flakes, salt and pepper.

2. Put the stuff into egg whites. Put into refrigerator till serving.

Nutritional information per serving:

Calories: 114

Fat: 9g

Protein: 6g

Carbohydrates: 1g

#15. Pimiento and Cheese Deviled Eggs Recipe

Total Prepare/ Cook Time: - 20 min.

Servings: 12

Ingredients:

6 large eggs (hard-cooked)

1/4 cup cheddar cheese, finely shredded

4 teaspoons pimiento, finely chopped

2 tablespoons mayonnaise

2 teaspoons Dijon mustard

2 teaspoons sweet onion, finely chopped

1 medium garlic clove, crumbled

Salt and pepper according to taste

Instructions:

1. Cut the eggs into halves and take out yolks. Mash yolks in a small bowl.

2. Mix 3 teaspoons pimiento, mayonnaise, cheese, onion, pepper, mustard and salt completely.

3. Put stuff into egg whites and drizzle with remaining pimiento. Put into refrigerator till serving.

Nutritional information per serving:

Calories: 66

Fat: 5g

Protein: 4g

Carbohydrates: 1g

#16. Special-Ingredients Stuffed Eggs Recipe

Total Prepare/ Cook Time: - 15 min.

Servings: 12

Ingredients:

6 large eggs (hard-cooked)

4 tablespoons goat cheese, crumbled

3 tablespoons pecans, finely chopped

2 tablespoons celery, finely chopped

3 tablespoons mayonnaise

2 tablespoons mango chutney

1/8 teaspoon pepper

1/4 teaspoon salt

Instructions:

1. Cut the eggs into halves and take out yolks. Mash yolks in a small bowl.

2. Mix 3 tablespoons goat cheese, mayonnaise, 2 tablespoons pecans, chutney, celery, pepper and salt completely.

3. Put stuff into egg whites and drizzle with remaining goat cheese and pecans. Put into refrigerator till serving.

Nutritional information per serving:

Calories: 97

Fat: 7g

Protein: 4g

Carbohydrates: 3g

#17. Fluffy-White Frosting Recipe

Total Prepare/ Cook Time: - 20 min.

Servings: 32

Ingredients:

4 egg whites

1 tablespoon water

Artificial sweetener equivalent to 1-1/3 cups sugar

1 teaspoon vanilla extract

1/2 teaspoon cream of tartar

Instructions:

1. Take a heatproof bowl, beat egg whites, water, artificial sweetener and cream of tartar until smooth.

2. Place over boiling water in a large saucepan over medium heat. Beating constantly for approx.3-4 minutes, then remove from heat and add vanilla.

3. Beat on high speed for approx. 7-8 minutes. Serve immediately.

Nutritional information per serving: 2 tablespoons

Calories: 35

Fat: trace

Protein: trace

Carbohydrates: 8g

#18. Swiss Oven Omelet Recipe

Total Prepare/ Cook Time: - 30 min.

Servings: 6

Ingredients:

2 cups red onion, finely chopped

1 tablespoon olive oil

Artificial sweetener equivalent to 2 teaspoons sugar

1/4 cup green onion, finely chopped

1/2 teaspoon thyme, dried

2 teaspoons Dijon mustard

6 eggs

1/4 teaspoon pepper

1/4 cup water

4 oz. Swiss cheese, cut into pieces

Instructions:

1. Take a large frying pan, mix red onion and artificial sweetener with spoon in olive oil and cook over medium heat for 10-12 minutes. Then take out 1/4 cup and put aside.

2. Now mix green onion, thyme and mustard into the frying pan and remove from the heat.

3. Take a bowl and beat eggs, pepper, water and salt then pour to the frying pan. Drizzle with 1/4 cup cheese.

4. Bake for approx. 15-18 minutes at 375 Fahrenheit. Topping with remaining onion mixture and cheese.

Nutritional information per serving:

Calories: 192

Fat: 12g

Protein: 12g

Carbohydrates: 8g

#19. Goat Cheese and Ham Omelet Recipe

Total Prepare/ Cook Time: - 20 min.

Servings: 1

Ingredients:

4 egg whites

1/8 teaspoon pepper

2 teaspoons water

1 slice deli ham, chopped

2 tablespoons onion, finely chopped

2 tablespoons goat cheese, crumbled

2 tablespoons green pepper, finely chopped

Fresh parsley, shredded

Instructions:

1. Take a small bowl, beat egg whites, pepper and water properly and mix with spoon in ham, onion and green pepper.

2. Grease a large frying pan with cooking spray, pour egg white mixture and heat up over medium heat.

3. When egg cooked completely then drizzle with goat cheese on one side of omelet. Fold omelet in half and drizzle with parsley.

4. Enjoy your delicious goat cheese and ham omelet with your family and friends.

Nutritional information per serving:

Calories: 143

Fat: 4g

Protein: 21g

Carbohydrates: 5g

DINNER EGG RECIPES

#20. Santa Fe Deviled Egg Recipe

Total Prepare/ Cook Time: - 15 min.

Servings: 2

Ingredients:

2 large eggs (hard-cooked)

1 tablespoon mayonnaise

1 tablespoon green chilies, chopped

Chipotle pepper in adobo sauce (1/2 teaspoon)

4 teaspoons salsa

1/8 teaspoon garlic salt

1-1/2 teaspoons green onion, thinly sliced

1 pitted ripe olive

Instructions:

1. Cut the eggs into halves and take out yolks. Mash yolks in a small bowl. Mix with spoon in mayonnaise, chipotle pepper, chilies and garlic salt.

2. Put stuff into egg whites. Drizzle with salsa, olive piece and onion. Put into refrigerator till serving.

Nutritional information per serving:

Calories: 111

Fat: 8g

Protein: 6g

Carbohydrates: 2g

#21. Bacon Cheddar Frittata Recipe

Total Prepare/ Cook Time: - 20 min.

Servings: 2

Ingredients:

3 eggs

1/2 cup milk

1 green onion, finely chopped

1 tablespoon melted butter

Small amount of pepper

1/4 teaspoon salt

1/2 cup cheddar cheese, cut into pieces

1 cooked bacon strip, crumbled

Instructions:

1. Take a medium bowl and beat the eggs, onion, milk, pepper, butter and salt well.

2. Grease the baking dish with cooking spray. Put the egg mixture into shallow 3-cups.

3. Drizzle with bacon and cheese. Bake for approx. 14-15 minutes at 400 Fahrenheit.

4. Enjoy the yummy Bacon Cheddar Frittata with your family and friends.

Nutritional information per serving:

Calories: 227

Fat: 14g

Protein: 22g

Carbohydrates: 5g

#22. Golden Sea Bass Recipe

Total Prepare/ Cook Time: - 25 min.

Servings: 8

Ingredients:

1 cup potato flakes, mashed

1 egg

1/4 teaspoon pepper

1 envelope Italian salad dressing mix

2 tablespoons melted butter

2 pounds sea bass fillets

Paprika

Instructions:

1. Take a medium bowl and mix potato flakes, pepper and dressing mix. Beat the egg in another bowl.

2. Dip fillets into egg and then grease with potato flake mixture.

3. Grease a large baking pan with cooking spray and put the egg mixture in single layer.

4. Drizzle with butter and paprika. Bake for approx. 15 minutes at 450 Fahrenheit.

Nutritional information per serving:

Calories: 180

Fat: 6g

Protein: 22g

Carbohydrates: 8g

#23. Basil Zucchini Pancakes Recipe

Total Prepare/ Cook Time: - 20 min.

Servings: 2

Ingredients:

1 cup zucchini, shredded

1 large egg

3 tablespoons baking mix

2 tablespoons cheddar cheese

1/8 teaspoon pepper

1/4 teaspoon basil, dried

1/8 teaspoon salt

Instructions:

1. Remove excess liquid from zucchini and put into colander to drain.

2. Take a small bowl and mix zucchini, baking mix, egg, pepper, cheese, basil and salt.

3. Grease a large skillet with cooking spray and put the egg mixture onto skillet.

4. Cook on both side for approx. 4-5 minutes over medium heat.

Nutritional information per serving:

Calories: 115

Fat: 6g

Protein: 6g

Carbohydrates: 9g

#24. Simple Lettuce Salad Recipe

Total Prepare/ Cook Time: - 10 min.

Servings: 2

Ingredients:

2 cups torn leaf lettuce

1 large egg, hard cooked and chopped

1 green onion, thinly sliced

1 teaspoon cider vinegar

2 tablespoons mayonnaise

1/8 teaspoon pepper

Instructions:

1. Take a small bowl and mix the lettuce, onion and egg.

2. Take another small bowl and whisk the mayonnaise, pepper and vinegar.

3. Put over the salad and mix them completely and enjoy it.

Nutritional information per serving:

Calories: 150

Fat: 14g

Protein: 4g

Carbohydrates: 3g

#25. Broccoli Fritters Recipe

Total Prepare/ Cook Time: - 25 min.

Servings: 6

Ingredients:

1 bunch broccoli, cut into florets

2 large lightly beaten eggs

2 lightly beaten egg whites

2 tablespoons all-purpose flour

1/3 cup parmesan cheese

1/2 teaspoon salt

1/2 teaspoon pepper

1/2 teaspoon garlic powder

2 tablespoons canola oil

Salsa

Instructions:

1. Put the broccoli in steamer basket then place in a small saucepan over 1 inch of water. Let the water comes to boil and steam broccoli for 3-4 minutes.

2. Chop the broccoli finely and put aside. Take a large bowl and mix eggs, egg whites, flour, cheese, pepper, garlic powder and salt. Mix with spoon in broccoli.

3. Take a large frying pan and heat up one tablespoon oil over medium heat. Put the egg and broccoli mixture into oil and press lightly. Cook for 4-5 minutes in batches.

4. Drain on paper towels and serve with salsa.

Nutritional information per serving:

1 serving= 2 Fritters

Calories: 129

Fat: 8g

Protein: 8g

Carbohydrates: 8g

#26. Shrimp Egg Recipe

Total Prepare/ Cook Time: - 30 min.

Servings: 4

Ingredients:

14 oz. suey vegetables, chopped and drained

1/2 pound cooked small shrimp, finely chopped

4 green onions, thinly sliced

4 large lightly beaten eggs

2 tablespoons canola oil

Green Pea Sauce:

2 cups water

1 teaspoon chicken bouillon granules

2 tablespoons cornstarch

1/2 cup frozen peas, thawed

1-1/2 teaspoons soy sauce (low-sodium)

Instructions:

1. Take a large bowl and mix suey vegetables, green onions and shrimp. Now mix with spoon in eggs.

2. Take a large frying pan and heat up 1 teaspoon oil over medium heat. Now put 1/4th part of the vegetable mixture into frying pan. Cook in batches.

3. Take a small saucepan and mix cornstarch and bouillon. Slowly mix in water and soy sauce. Left the mixture until it comes to boil. Cook for approx. 3 minutes. Now mix with spoon in peas. Heat up for small time. Serve with Cooked egg.

Nutritional information per serving:

Calories: 242

Fat: 13g

Protein: 20g

Carbohydrates: 9g

#27. Oven Denver Omelet Recipe

Total Prepare/ Cook Time: - 30 min.

Servings: 4-6

Ingredients:

8 large eggs

4 oz. cheddar cheese, cut into pieces

1/2 cup half-and-half cream

1 cup fully cooked ham, finely chopped

1/4 cup green pepper, finely chopped

1/4 cup onion, finely chopped

Instructions:

1. Take a large bowl and beat eggs and cream completely. Mix with spoon in cheese, ham, onion and green pepper. Grease a large baking dish and pour the mixture over it.

2. Bake for approx. 25 minutes at 400 Fahrenheit. Enjoy the delicious Oven Denver Omelet with your family and friend.

Nutritional information per serving:

Calories: 235

Fat: 16g

Protein: 17g

Carbohydrates: 4g

#28. Corned Beef Omelet Recipe

Total Prepare/ Cook Time: - 20 min.

Servings: 4

Ingredients:

6 large eggs

2 green onions, thinly sliced

2 tablespoons butter

1/2 cup cheddar cheese

1/4 cup milk

1 cup cooked corned beef

Small amount of pepper

Instructions:

1. Take a large frying pan and fry onions in butter. Now take a large bowl and beat eggs and milk and put over onions and cook over medium heat.

2. When the eggs cooked completely, drizzle with corned beef, pepper and cheese.

3. Take away from the heat and let stand for 2-3 minutes, cut into pieces.

4. Enjoy your delicious corned beef omelet with your family and friends.

Nutritional information per serving:

Calories: 291

Fat: 23g

Protein: 18g

Carbohydrates: 2g

#29. Parmesan Zucchini Omelet Recipe

Total Prepare/ Cook Time: - 15 min.

Servings: 2

Ingredients:

3 large eggs

1/2 cup zucchini, thinly sliced

2 onions, thinly sliced

2 tablespoons butter

3 tablespoons water

1/4 cup seeded tomato, finely chopped

1/8 teaspoon thyme, dried

3 tablespoons parmesan cheese, shredded

1/8 teaspoon salt

Small amount of pepper

Instructions:

1. Take a large frying pan and fry onion and zucchini in butter. Take a small bowl and mix lightly beaten eggs, thyme, water, pepper and salt and pour over vegetables.

2. Cook over medium heat. When eggs are completely cooked drizzle with cheese and tomato. Put 4-6 in. away from the heat for approx. 2 minutes or until cheese is melted.

3. Before serving cut into two halves and enjoy this yummy recipe with your family.

Nutritional information per serving:

Calories: 258

Fat: 21g

Protein: 13g

Carbohydrates: 4g

APPETIZERS

#30. Halloween Eyeball Appetizer Recipe

Total Prepare/ Cook Time: - 40 min.

Servings: 12

Ingredients:

6 eggs

2 tablespoons red food coloring

3 cups hot water

1/3 cup mayonnaise

1 tablespoon white vinegar

1/4 cup green onion, finely chopped

2 teaspoons Dijon mustard

2 tablespoons fresh cilantro, crumbled

12 slices of ripe olives

1 teaspoon ketchup

Instructions:

1. Take a large saucepan and put eggs in one single layer. Add cold water upto 1 in. of the pan. Let the water comes to boil over high heat.

2. Just take away from heat and let for 12 minutes, put into chilled water until completely cooled. Gradually crack eggs.

3. Take a large bowl and mix 3 cups hot water, vinegar and food coloring. Add eggs and left for 30 minutes. Take out eggs from water.

4. Cut eggs into halves and put yolks into small bowl. Put egg whites aside and mash yolks completely then mix with spoon in mayonnaise, cilantro, mustard and onions.

5. Stuff yolk mixture into egg whites. Put olive slice on each with ketchup. Put into refrigerator till serving.

Nutritional information per serving:

Calories: 83

Fat: 7g

Protein: 3g

Carbohydrates: 1g

#31. Holiday Appetizer Puffs Recipe

Total Prepare/ Cook Time: - 45 min.

Servings: 16

Ingredients:

1 cup water

1/2 cup butter

4 eggs

1 cup all-purpose flour

1/2 teaspoon salt

FILLING:

8 oz. softened cream cheese

6 oz. crabmeat without cartilage

1/4 cup mayonnaise

1/2 cup Swiss cheese, shredded

1 teaspoon garlic salt

1 tablespoon chives, minced

1/4 teaspoon pepper

1 teaspoon Worcestershire sauce

Instructions:

1. Take a small pan add water, butter and salt and heat up over medium heat, left until the mixture comes to boil.

2. Add flour into mixture and take away from heat and stand for 5-6 minutes. Mix eggs into mixture and beat until the mixture becomes smooth.

3. Grease baking sheets and put the mixture with teaspoon onto baking sheets. Bake for approx. 30 minutes at 400 Fahrenheit.

4. Put onto wire racks and Cut a slit into puff so as the steam should escape from puffs.

5. Take a small bowl then mix mayonnaise and cream cheese completely. Mix with spoon in remaining filling. Just put the filling into puffs before serving.

Nutritional information per serving:

1 serving = 3 puffs

Calories: 195

Fat: 16g

Protein: 7g

Carbohydrates: 7g

#32. Stuffed Shrimp Appetizer Recipe

Total Prepare/ Cook Time: - 35 min.

Servings: 20

Ingredients:

20 large shrimp, uncooked

1 large beaten egg

1/2 cup soft bread crumbs

1/2 teaspoon fresh lemon juice

1 tablespoon mayonnaise

1/4 teaspoon pepper

1/4 teaspoon seasoning blend (salt-free)

Small amount of cayenne pepper

1/8 teaspoon oregano, dried

2 tablespoon parmesan cheese, grated

6 oz. lump crabmeat, drained

1 teaspoon paprika

Instructions:

1. Butterfly each shrimp along outside curve. Take a large ungreased baking pan and put butterflied portion into baking pan.

2. Take a small bowl and mix the egg, mayonnaise, bread crumbs, lemon juice and seasoning. Mix with spoon in crab.

3. Put 1 tablespoon of mixture over each shrimp and drizzle with paprika and cheese.

4. Bake for approx. 10-12 minutes at 350 Fahrenheit. Serve immediately.

Nutritional information per serving:

Calories: 36

Fat: 1g

Protein: 5g

Carbohydrates: 1g

#33. Barbecue Sauce Meatballs Recipe

Total Prepare/ Cook Time: - 45 min.

Servings: 18

Ingredients:

1 large beaten egg

1 tablespoon onion, finely chopped

1/4 teaspoon pepper

1/2 teaspoon salt

1 cup crisp rice cereal, crushed

1 pound ground beef, crumbled

SAUCE:

3 tablespoons ketchup

1/4 cup packed brown sugar

1/8 teaspoon ground nutmeg

1 teaspoon prepared mustard

Instructions:

1. Take a large bowl and mix the egg, onion, salt, pepper and 3/4 cup cereal. Now put beef over mixture and mix them completely.

2. Take a small bowl and mix the remaining ingredients for making sauce. Pour 2 tablespoons sauce to meat mixture and make them like 1-1/2 in. balls.

3. Grease the rack with cooking spray and put the meatballs over it in a shallow baking pan. Pour the remaining sauce and drizzle with remaining cereal.

4. Bake for 25 minutes at 400 Fahrenheit. Enjoy the delicious Barbecue sauce meatballs with your family.

Nutritional information per serving:

1 serving = 1 meatball

Calories: 74

Fat: 3g

Protein: 5g

Carbohydrates: 5g

#34. Sweet 'n' Spicy Meatballs Recipe

Total Prepare/ Cook Time: - 40 min.

Servings: 48

Ingredients:

1 lightly beaten egg

2 pound bulk spicy pork sausage

1 cup red wine vinegar

1 cup packed brown sugar

1 cup ketchup

1 teaspoon ground ginger

1 tablespoon soy sauce

Instructions:

1. Take a large bowl and mix sausage and egg well. Make them like 1 in. ball shape.

2. Grease the rack with cooking spray and put the meatballs over it in a shallow baking pan.

3. Bake for 20 minutes approx. at 400 Fahrenheit. While the egg sausage baking take a small saucepan and mix the remaining ingredients.

4. Wait till the mixture comes to boil. Slow down the heat and cook over low heat.

5. Put the meatballs into small crock pot. Add the sauce and coat them. Till serving keep warm on low.

Nutritional information per serving:

1 serving = 1 meatball

Calories: 64

Fat: 4g

Protein: 2g

Carbohydrates: 6g

#35. Hop-To-It Deviled Eggs Recipe

Total Prepare/ Cook Time: - 20 min.

Servings: 12

Ingredients:

6 large eggs (hard-cooked)

1 tablespoon sweet pickle relish

1/4 cup mayonnaise

1/2 teaspoon honey mustard

Salt and pepper to taste

12 chives

1/4 cup alfalfa sprouts

1/4 cup sunflower kernels (candy-coated)

Instructions:

1. Cut the eggs into halves and take out yolks. Mash yolks in a small bowl. Mix mayonnaise, mustard, relish, salt and pepper well. Put the stuff into egg whites.

2. Drizzle sprouts and put the ends of chive into each egg form like handle.

3. Put into refrigerator before serving and garnish with sunflower kernels.

Nutritional information per serving:

Calories: 93

Fat: 7g

Protein: 4g

Carbohydrates: 3g

#36. Healthy Cheese Stuffed Mushrooms Recipe

Total Prepare/ Cook Time: - 15 min.

Servings: 8

Ingredients:

1 finely chopped egg (hard-cooked)

1/4 cup Swiss cheese, shredded

2 tablespoons melted butter

4-1/2 teaspoons seasoned bread crumbs

8 large fresh mushrooms

1/4 teaspoon garlic, minced

1/8 teaspoon salt

Instructions:

1. Take a small bowl and mix egg, cheese, bread crumbs, garlic, 1 tablespoon butter and salt. Put aside.

2. Remove stems from mushrooms and put into hollow baking sheet greased with cooking spray. Coated with remaining butter.

3. Heat for approx. 5 minutes, 4 in. away from the direct heat contact. Put the cheese mixture over it. Heat for 3-4 minutes, away from direct heat.

4. Enjoy the delicious Healthy Cheese Stuffed Mushrooms with your family.

Nutritional information per serving:

Calories: 59

Fat: 5g

Protein: 3g

Carbohydrates: 2g

#37. Fried Cheese Ravioli Recipe

Total Prepare/ Cook Time: - 35 min.

Servings: 45

Ingredients:

9 oz. chilled cheese ravioli

2 cups seasoned bread crumbs

2 large eggs

3 teaspoons basil, dried

1/2 cup parmesan cheese, shredded

1/2 cup canola oil

1 cup warmed marinara sauce

Instructions:

1. Cook ravioli according to directions given at the package. Beat the eggs in a small bowl.

2. Take another small bowl and mix cheese, bread crumbs and basil. First dip ravioli in eggs then in bread crumbs mixture.

3. Take a large frying pan and heat 1/4 cup oil over medium heat. Fry ravioli for 1-2 minutes on each side in batches and when it cooked then drain it.

4. Drizzle with extra cheese and enjoy with marinara sauce.

Nutritional information per serving:

Calories: 37

Fat: 1g

Protein: 2g

Carbohydrates: 5g

#38. Chicks-On-the-Ranch Deviled Eggs Recipe

Total Prepare/ Cook Time: - 25 min.

Servings: 6

Ingredients:

6 large eggs (hard-cooked)

1/4 cup ranch salad dressing

1/4 cup parmesan cheese, cut into pieces

5 carrot chips

1 teaspoon Dijon mustard

12 capers

Fresh dill springs

Small amount of pepper

Instructions:

1. Cut the top third from each egg and take out yolks. Mash yolks in a small bowl.

2. Mix salad dressing, cheese, pepper and mustard well. Put stuff into egg whites.

3. Cut 12 small triangles and 12 feet for beaks from carrot chips. Slowly press the capers into the filling and beaks also.

4. Put feet in front of chicks. Put into refrigerator before serving.

Nutritional information per serving:

Calories: 145

Fat: 12g

Protein: 8g

Carbohydrates: 2g

#39. Garlic-Herb Mini Quiches Recipe

Total Prepare/ Cook Time: - 25 min.

Servings: 45

Ingredients:

6-1/2 oz. garlic herb spreadable cheese (low-fat)

2 large eggs

1/4 cup milk (fat-free)

3 package of chilled miniature phyllo tart shells

2 tablespoons fresh parsley, minced

Instructions:

1. Take a small bowl and mix the spreadable cheese, eggs and milk. Take a uncoated baking sheet and put tart shells into it.

2. Fill each tart shells with 2 teaspoons mixture and drizzle with parsley.

3. Bake for 12-14 minutes at 350 Fahrenheit or until the shells baked completely.

4. Serve immediately.

Nutritional information per serving:

Calories: 31

Fat: 2g

Protein: 1g

Carbohydrates: 2g

SNACKS

#40. Swiss Seafood Canapés Recipe

Total Prepare/ Cook Time: - 25 min.

Servings: 48

Ingredients:

6 oz. small shrimp, washed and drained

6 oz. chilled crabmeat

1 cup Swiss cheese, cut into pieces

2 large eggs, (hard-cooked) finely chopped

1/4 cup mayonnaise

1/4 cup celery, finely chopped

2 green onions, finely chopped

1/4 cup French salad dressing

1 loaf snack rye bread

Salt to taste

Instructions:

1. Take a large bowl and mix all the ingredients except snack rye bread. Now take an ungreased baking sheet and put bread on it. Heat for approx. 2 minutes, 5 in. away from direct heat.

2. Cut the bread into slices and put 1 tablespoonful of seafood mixture on each bread slice.

3. Again heat for approx. 4 minutes, 3-4 in. away from direct heat.

4. Enjoy the yummy Swiss Seafood Canapés with your family.

Nutritional information per serving:

Calories: 57

Fat: 3g

Protein: 3g

Carbohydrates: 5g

#41. Party Chicken Spread Recipe

Total Prepare/ Cook Time: - 25 min.

Servings: 12

Ingredients:

8 oz. softened cream cheese

2 tablespoons fresh lemon juice

1/4 cup mayonnaise

1/4 teaspoon ground ginger

1/8 teaspoon pepper

1/2 teaspoon salt

1/8 teaspoon hot pepper sauce

2 cups cooked chicken breast, finely chopped

2 large finely chopped eggs, (hard-cooked)

1/4 cup green onions, thinly sliced

Diced pimientos

Snack rye bread

Instructions:

1. Take a large bowl and mix cream cheese, mayonnaise, lemon juice, salt, pepper, ground ginger and hot pepper sauce well.

2. Mix with spoon in chicken, eggs and green onions. Give the shape of 8-in. x 2-in. log and garnish with onions and pimientos.

3. Put into refrigerator for some time and remove from refrigerator 15 minutes before serving.

4. Enjoy this delicious recipe with bread.

Nutritional information per serving:

Calories: 100

Fat: 5g

Protein: 10g

Carbohydrates: 3g

#42. Spiced Party Peanuts Recipe

Total Prepare/ Cook Time: - 30 min.

Servings: 12

Ingredients:

1 egg white

1 teaspoon water

3 cups roasted peanuts, dry and unsalted

1 teaspoon ground cinnamon

Artificial sweetener equivalent to 1 tablespoon sugar

1/4 teaspoon salt

1/2 teaspoon cayenne pepper

1/4 teaspoon ground coriander

1/4 teaspoon ground cumin

Instructions:

1. Take a large bowl, beat egg white and water completely. Pour into peanuts.

2. Mix spices and artificial sweetener then add to peanut mixture and stir slowly.

3. Take an uncoated large baking pan and put the mixture into it. Bake for 22-25 minutes at 325 Fahrenheit. Put onto wire rack for cooling.

Nutritional information per serving:

Calories: 220

Fat: 18g

Protein: 9g

Carbohydrates: 9g

#43. Artichoke Rye Toasts Recipe

Total Prepare/ Cook Time: - 40 min.

Servings: 12

Ingredients:

Chilled butter flavored spray

4 egg whites

24 slices snack rye bread

14 oz. artichoke hearts, drained and finely chopped

1/4 teaspoon paprika

1/8 teaspoon cayenne pepper

1/4 cup cheddar cheese, cut into pieces

1/4 cup parmesan cheese, grated

Instructions:

1. Take uncoated baking sheets and place the bread over it and spritz with butter flavored spray.

2. Take a small bowl and mix the artichoke, cayenne and cheeses well. Take another small bowl, beat egg whites completely and put into artichoke mixture.

3. Put over bread and drizzle with paprika. Bake for approx. 12-14 minutes at 400 Fahrenheit. Serve immediately.

Nutritional information per serving:

Calories: 78

Fat: 2g

Protein: 5g

Carbohydrates: 9g

#44. Sugar-Free Spiced Pecans Recipe

Total Prepare/ Cook Time: - 30 min.

Servings: 20

Ingredients:

1 large egg white

3 teaspoons ground cinnamon

Artificial sweetener equivalent to 1/2 cup sugar

1 pound pecan halves

1/2 teaspoon salt

Instructions:

1. Take a large bowl and beat egg white completely. Add pecans coat them.

2. Now mix the artificial sweetener, salt and cinnamon and put into nut mixture.

3. Grease a large baking pan with cooking spray and put the mixture into it.

4. Bake for approx. 20 minutes at 325 Fahrenheit. Wait until it cools down.

Nutritional information per serving:

Calories: 161

Fat: 16g

Protein: 2g

Carbohydrates: 4g

DESSERTS

#45. Crunchy Macaroons Recipe

Total Prepare/ Cook Time: - 35 min.

Servings: 12

Ingredients:

2 egg whites

Artificial sweetener equivalent to 3 tablespoons sugar

1-1/2 cups crisp rice cereal

1/8 teaspoon almond extract

1-1/4 cups flaked coconut

Instructions:

1. Take a small bowl and mix all the ingredients well. Then make them into 1-1/2 in. mounds on parchment paper lined baking sheets with wet fingers.

2. Bake for approx. 25 minutes at 300 Fahrenheit. When it completely baked then put onto wire rack to cool.

Nutritional information per serving:

1 serving = 2 cookies

Calories: 76

Fat: 3g

Protein: 2g

Carbohydrates: 10g

#46. Honey Almond Nougats Recipe

Total Prepare/ Cook Time: - 30 min.

Servings: 45

Ingredients:

2 egg whites

1/2 cup honey

2 teaspoons cornstarch

1-1/2 teaspoon butter

Artificial sweetener equivalent to 2/3 cup superfine sugar

2 cups ground almonds

1 cup almonds, finely chopped

1 teaspoon ground cinnamon

Instructions:

1. Take a large bowl and coated with butter. Take a large saucepan and mix cornstarch, artificial sweetener and honey. Cook over medium heat and boil for 2 minutes.

2. Put the beaten egg whites into mixer, running on high speed then pour hot artificial sweetener mixture and then beat for 10 more minutes on high.

3. Put in ground almonds and cinnamon then place to a bowl. Make them into 1 in. balls. Garnish with chopped almonds.

Nutritional information per serving:

Calories: 66

Fat: 4g

Protein: 2g

Carbohydrates: 8g

#47. Crackle Cookies Recipe

Total Prepare/ Cook Time: - 30 min.

Servings: 18

Ingredients:

2 tablespoons canola oil

1 large egg

1 oz. melted chocolate, unsweetened and cooled

Artificial sweetener equivalent to 1/2 cup sugar

1/2 teaspoon vanilla extract

1/2 cup all-purpose flour

1/8 teaspoon salt

1/2 teaspoon baking powder

Confectioner's sugar

Instructions:

1. Take a bowl combine vanilla, oil, chocolate and artificial sweetener completely. Take another bowl and mix baking powder, flour and salt, slowly beat into artificial sweetener mixture. Put into refrigerator.

2. Heat up oven to 350 Fahrenheit. Give them shape into 1 in. balls then roll in confectioner's sugar.

3. Put 2 in. away on coated baking sheets and bake for 11-12 minutes. After baking, put onto wire rack for cooling.

4. Enjoy this delicious crackle cookies with your friends and family.

Nutritional information per serving:

Calories: 60

Fat: 3g

Protein: 1g

Carbohydrates: 9g

#48. Bake-Sale Lemon Bars Recipe

Total Prepare/ Cook Time: - 45 min.

Servings: 48

Ingredients:

3/4 cup butter

3 large eggs

2/3 cup confectioner's sugar

1-1/2 cups all-purpose flour

1/4 cup fresh lemon juice

Artificial sweetener equivalent to 1/2 cup sugar

Instructions:

1. Take a large bowl and combine butter and confectioner's sugar completely.

2. Put into 1-1/2 cups flour and mix them properly. Put onto large coated baking pan. Bake for 15-20 minutes at 350 Fahrenheit.

3. At the same time take a small bowl and beat eggs, lemon juice, remaining flour and artificial sweetener then pour over hot crust.

4. Again bake for 20-22 minutes then put over wire rack for cooling. Put into refrigerator before serving.

Nutritional information per serving:

Calories: 77

Fat: 3g

Protein: 1g

Carbohydrates: 10g

#49. Prune Pecan Cookies Recipe

Total Prepare/ Cook Time: - 25 min.

Servings: 24

Ingredients:

1 large egg

Artificial sweetener equivalent to 1/2 cup sugar

7 pitted dried plums

1/2 teaspoon baking soda

1 cup all-purpose flour

Salt to taste

24 pecan halves

Instructions:

1. Blend egg and plums completely then pour into a medium bowl.

2. Combine artificial sweetener, flour, salt and baking soda into plum mixture and mix them well.

3. Grease the baking sheets and put the mixture onto it. Drizzle with pecan half on each cookie.

4. Bake for approx. 15 minutes at 350 Fahrenheit. After baking put onto wire rack for cooling.

5. Enjoy this yummy recipe with your family.

Nutritional information per serving:

Calories: 54

Fat: 1g

Protein: 1g

Carbohydrates: 9g